CBD O

Your Natural Choice for Pain Relief and Living A Healthier and Happier Life

By: Jim Russlan

© **Copyright 2018 - All rights reserved.**

The content contained within this book may not be reproduced, duplicated or transmitted without direct written permission from the author or the publisher.

Under no circumstances will any blame or legal responsibility be held against the publisher or author for any damages, reparation, or monetary loss due to the information contained within this book. Either directly or indirectly.

Legal Notice:

This book is copyright protected. This book is only for personal use. You cannot amend, distribute, sell, use, quote or paraphrase any part, or the content within this book, without the consent of the author or publisher.

Disclaimer Notice:

Please note the information contained within this document is for educational and entertainment purposes only. All effort has been executed to present accurate, up to date and reliable information. No warranties of any kind are declared or implied. Readers acknowledge that the author is not engaging in the rendering of legal, financial, medical or professional advice. The content within this book has been derived from various sources. Please consult a licensed professional before attempting any techniques in this book.

By reading this document, the reader agrees that under no circumstances is the author responsible for any losses, which are incurred as a result of the use of information contained within this document, including, but not limited to errors, omissions, or inaccuracies.

BONUS!

First of all, I wish to congratulate you on making a choice that you want to be proactive and to do something about your situation.

Click here for free access!

I am always happy to help such a person and for that I would like to make you an exclusive offer to join an exclusive service which will send you ways and tips for improving your life and you will also be among the first people to find out about my latest books on different areas of health and pain free living. That's not even the best part. By signing up you will receive an additional resource about CBD oil completely free of charge. If all of this sounds good to you, then it can be yours by following the link above for FREE access.

TABLE OF CONTENTS:

Introduction..1
Chapter 1: Introduction To CBD Oil....................................2
Chapter 2: Health Benefits Of CBD Oil...............................8
Chapter 3: How to – CBD..19
Chapter 4: Possible Side Effects with CBD oil................28
Chapter 5: Is CBD Oil Legal?..33
Chapter 6: Where to Buy CBD Oil/Costs.........................45
Chapter 7: Success Stories Related to CBD....................50
Conclusion..60

Introduction

CBD oil seems to be the new craze. I am sure you've heard about it, whether online, on TV, or maybe even someone you know has given it a try. Everyone's talking about it, but only a few actually seem to know what it is exactly. Does it get you high? Is it a "drug"? Is it legal? Where can I get CBD oil?

In "CBD Oil for Pain, Your natural choice for pain relief and living a healthier and happier lifestyle," we will take a look at what CBD oil exactly is – the science behind it, how it differs from its "cousin" THC or tetrahydrocannabinol, and how it affects our human body. We will look at what it does for you– all of CBD oil's health benefits that range from pain relief, to help with sleep, and even helping reduce seizures in children with epilepsy. You will really get to see why so many people are taking CBD oil.

We will take a look at the many ways to use CBD oil, and how to do so successfully and correctly. We're going to find out where CBD oil is legal (I am sure no one wants any trouble with the law!) Of course, you will also want to know where to get CBD oil, how much to get, how much it costs, etc.

We will look at any possible side effects – what exactly CBD oil can do to you that you might not like. We will also learn about real people who had real-life success with CBD oil.

Chapter 1: Introduction To CBD Oil

CBD or "cannabidiol" has been discovered around the 1940s. Dr. Roger Adams discovered CBD at the University of Illinois – more than twenty years before THC (the other major constituent in marijuana) was discovered. The entire structure of CBD was not elucidated until 1963. It has been used medicinally since the 19th century. It is said that Queen Victoria, Queen of the United Kingdom and Ireland from 1837 to 1901, used CBD to treat menstrual cramps. Cannabis itself has been used medicinally since as early as 1400-2000 BC.

William Osler is said to have created the first program pushing for the medicinal use of cannabis. Osler, often referred to as the "Father of Modern Medicine," believed cannabis could help with headaches. In 1937, cannabis was on its way to being used for industrial and medicinal purposes with the "Marijuana Tax Act." Cannabis was then criminalized in 1969, and the act was ruled unconstitutional. For quite some time, the research in the United States regarding the medicinal benefits of cannabis stopped.

In 1998, a company called GW Pharmaceuticals, based in Cambridge, United Kingdom began growing cannabis in order to use it for clinical trials. The goal was to produce CBD-rich plants and in turn, produce a medicine that had little to no psychoactive effects. A "CBD-rich" plant is considered to have at least 4 percent CBD (dry weight). The CBD-rich plants not only countered the psychoactive effects of THC but also had their own benefits.

GW Pharmaceuticals was given access to HortaPharm, a Dutch seed company's genetic library.

CBD is a naturally occurring cannabinoid. In hemp plants there are at least 130 cannabinoids - CBD is one of them and takes up to 40 percent of the plant's extract. When it was first discovered, it was not thought to be pharmaceutically active

CBD oil is taken from the flowers, stems, leaves or buds (resin glands) of marijuana (cannabis) or taken from hemp. It is commonly thought that CBD taken from marijuana is of better quality and concentration because it contains complementary cannabinoids. The flowers are going to be the most valuable due to their density, creating a full spectrum oil. Full spectrum CBD oil of high quality is often made with only the female flowers.

Hemp is a fibrous, industrial form of cannabis. Hemp has little tiny buds and a THC (tetrahydrocannabinol) level of 0.3 percent or less. CBD oil usually contains another type of oil such as MCT oil. THC is what gets you high, or produces the euphoric and intoxicating feelings. CBD oil will not get you "high," because it contains little to no THC.

Oddly enough, our bodies actually make their own cannabinoids and have a system to make them work together properly. For example, you should think of cannabinoids as little soldiers fighting along in your body. It is their job to make sure everything is balanced inside. Every living thing with a vertebrate has an endocannabinoid system (ECS). It is the endocannabinoid system that makes the cannabinoids or "soldiers."

The endocannabinoid system is still something many are unaware of. It is newly discovered within the animal and human body. The endocannabinoid system has very specific duties, much like our nervous system and immune system. The endocannabinoid system, as stated, is in charge of maintaining balance in the body, along with regulating homeostasis. It does things like regulating our mood, memory, pain perception, sleep, motor control, appetite, and more. The endocannabinoid system does so by producing the cannabinoids or "soldiers."

As we grow older, our endocannabinoid system begins to wear out – much like everything else within our bodies. As this happens, the endocannabinoid system starts to have trouble maintaining balance. Fewer cannabinoids are made, and you can even become cannabinoid deficient. The endocannabinoid system can also be disrupted if a person is sick, has a disease or is injured.

Unfortunately, once the body begins to run low on cannabinoids, there is not typically a "natural" way to get more. In fact, the last time you got cannabinoids was from your mother's milk during infancy (that is if you were breastfed). You probably are not going to have access to "mother's milk" at this stage in your life, so what gives? This is where cannabis/hemp plant comes into play.

Grown from the soil, CBD is the most populous of more than 100 various phyto-cannabinoids (Phyto means plant) that are within the cannabis/hemp plant. Plant-based cannabinoids stimulate your endocannabinoid system naturally by reinforcing it. In other terms, these cannabinoids or "plant soldiers" stimulate the body's natural defenses, which soothe your ailment. This allows the body to rebalance. Having an out of balance body can surface in many forms such as having chronic anxiety.

The best part of plant-based cannabinoids is that they are completely natural, given to us from the earth. They are not man-made, artificial, mixed with chemicals or physically addictive.

CBD works by exerting itself through several pathways. One site is the system of receptors found in the central and peripheral nervous systems, brain, muscle, fat and immune cells, called the endocannabinoid system. Although THC activates the endocannabinoid system stronger, the way CBD acts is more complex. Both constituents bind themselves to CB in the endocannabinoid receptor. CBD likely inhibits the release of glutamate, which is an excitatory neurotransmitter. The CB receptor is in charge of maintaining normal brain activity, such as protecting against seizures.

It is the CBD's interactions in the endocannabinoid system that counteracts the effects of THC, which are physiological and psychological. CBD also increases anandamide, an endocannabinoid. Anandamide has anti-inflammatory effects. Additionally, there is a biochemical target of CBD that is the TRP (transient receptor potential) class of channels. This affects calcium levels in the cell and can increase calcium levels in other cells as well.

The signaling of the 5HT-1A serotonin receptor is increased by CBD. Serotonin is found in the body, and it regulates the mood. What the CBD does is decrease anxiety. It protects the brain from oxidative stress, inflammation and increases levels of adenosine. Adenosine is a neurotransmitter and molecule that helps with sleep regulation and energy creation. A serotonin dysfunction is often due to depression or a number of other disorders.

In simpler terms, CBD helps the body with emotional and physical stress due to changes in the immediate environment by maintaining homeostasis.

There is a whole-plant CBD-rich oil and a single-molecule CBD. Single-molecule CBD is going to be less therapeutically effective. It lacks important secondary cannabinoids and other medicinal compounds.

CBD products typically fall into three categories. Crystalline isolate, which contains zero THC; unrefined full spectrum, which contains some THC but less than 0.3 percent, along with CBN and CBG; and full spectrum, which contains some THC but less than 0.3 percent.

Crystalline isolate has the appearance of salt crystals. The benefit is they have no taste and they do not contain any THC. The negative side of crystalline isolate is that it has no plant nutrients, making it a weak product. Essentially you need to consume a lot of the product to feel its CBD effects.
Unrefined full spectrum is very thick, cloudy and dark. The THC in unrefined full spectrum products amplifies the CBD effects. Unrefined full spectrum also has many other plant nutrients and cannabinoids such as CBN,

CBG, CBDV, terpenes, omega 3, omega 6, omega 9 and plant sterols. Unrefined full spectrum can be called "rick system style," meaning it is dark, raw and full of nutrients. However, with unrefined full spectrum, there is a certain ammount of THC present. Unrefined full spectrum can also have an earthy, unpleasant taste. It is important to get an unrefined full-spectrum product that has been properly flavored by the company who makes it.

Full spectrum oil is gold or see-through, to clear. The benefit of full spectrum products is that it is less refined than crystalline iodine, but has some THC as well. The THC helps with the CBD effects, making the product more effective. This is sometimes called the "entourage effect." Full spectrum products can also taste unpleasant, so again it is important to get a full spectrum product that has been properly flavored.

CBD oil has continued to gain popularity since the legalization of recreational marijuana in Colorado and Washington in 2012. Since then, several other states have also legalized recreational marijuana use, only adding to the popularity of CBD oil. Today, recreational marijuana use is legal in California, Alaska, Colorado, Maine, Oregon, Vermont, Massachusetts, Nevada, Washington and Washington DC.

In the past several years, CBD has continued to gain momentum in the health and wellness community. This is in part due to scientific studies proving the amazing benefits and potential that CBD contains.

Chapter 2: Health Benefits Of CBD Oil

CBD is just one of 100+ cannabinoids in cannabis. It has numerous health benefits including pain relief, help with epilepsy and help with sleeping problems. CBD oil can be used in treating cancer patients and much, much more.

Additionally, CBD is non-psychoactive, so you are not going to get "high" when consuming it. This makes it safer and more appealing to those worried about the mind-altering effects that THC can have.

Pain relief is one of the most highly regarded health benefits of CBD oil due to its analgesic effects. Apparently, CBD interacts with brain receptors and the immune system; this alleviates pain and reduces inflammation. Several studies have been conducted proving that CBD reduces inflammation within mice and rats.

Chronic inflammation is a large problem in our society that leads to many non-infectious diseases including cancer, Alzheimer's, heart disease, and autoimmune diseases, to name a few. A healthy diet and lifestyle is going to do wonders with chronic inflammation, but when a person is already doing both, along with getting good sleep and exercise, CBD oil can be an added bonus on top. Research has proven that CBD oil has the ability to reduce chronic inflammation that can lead to a disease.

More technically, CBD has the ability to blunt Th1 and Th2 dominance

In a study with rats with asthma, Th1 (TNF-a and IL-6) and Th2 (IL-4, IL-5, Il-13) responses were reduced after being treated with CBD.

CBD decreased the release and production of inflammatory cytokines like Th1 (IFN-gamma, TNF-alpha, and IL-6), Th2 (IL-4) and IL-8.

CBD has the ability to suppress Th17 dominance, meaning it can help with Th-17-dominant autoimmune diseases.

More anti-inflammatory mechanisms CBD has include reducing the mobilization and growth of neutrophils and reducing the inflammatory Macrophage Inflammatory Protein-1 (MIP-1 beta, MIP-1 alpha)

Studies show that CBD is an effective pain-relief treatment that causes no negative side effects in patients. Those who particularly suffer from fibromyalgia and multiple sclerosis can find pain relief in CBD oil. It is recommended for those with multiple sclerosis, to take a combination of CBD and THC. It will effectively treat muscle tightness, sleep disturbances, loss of bladder control (urinary incontinence), and pain.

CBD oil can be particularly helpful to those with rheumatoid arthritis; this is due to its anti-inflammatory effects. The CBD can help with swelling, joint pain, disease progression, and decrease joint destruction – this can lead to better quality of sleep. No negative side effects were discovered.

CBD oil can even prevent nervous system degeneration. The best part of CBD oil is that it does not allow one to develop a tolerance or become dependent on it like many opioids do. CBD oil is a wonderful choice for those who are looking to stay away from highly addictive opioids.

Epilepsy is another major thing that CBD oil can help with. Epilepsy causes excessive and abnormal brain cell activity; due to this, disturbance seizures occur. There have been many major newsworthy cases over the years that have brought attention to CBD oil for its anti-seizure properties.

More recently there have been studies done to back up these cases, showing that CBD oil is actually effective with epilepsy. Specifically, there is one form of epilepsy, Dravet Syndrome, which can be treated effectively with CBD oil. Dravet Syndrome is an uncommon form of epilepsy that is often induced by fever. Those with Dravet Syndrome who participated in the study conducted by The New England Journal of Medicine, and experienced reduced seizures. In this placebo-controlled, randomized, double-blind study, a median seizure frequency dropped by 38.9 percent.

In another survey that included children and their parents, 84 percent of the parents reported back that their children's seizure frequency reduced by 84 percent. These kids also experienced elevated mood, better sleep, and increased alertness. The only side effects were fatigue and drowsiness.

In addition, after three months of treatment with CBD oil, 39 percent of the kids had more than 50 percent reduction in their seizures.

CBD oil is also effective in treating some mental health conditions, most commonly anxiety. One study showed that, in particular, CBD oil can help with social anxiety disorder, post-traumatic stress disorder (PTSD) and obsessive-compulsive disorder. It also helps with the fear of public speaking.

Depression is another mental health condition that CBD oil can help with. It has been shown to do so by enhancing glutamate cortical signaling and serotonergic cortical signaling. Those with depression have a lack of both of those forms of cortical signaling. According to the Anxiety and Depression Association of America, anxiety affects 18 percent of the U.S. population, while 6 percent of the U.S. population is affected by depression.

CBD and schizophrenia

Schizophrenia is a complex and serious disease. This disease is most commonly managed with prescription medications and therapy. Unfortunately, many of the medications have negative side effects. CBD oil has been shown to lessen hallucinations in those with schizophrenia.

A March 2015 review stated that CBD oil is a harmless, effective and well-tolerated treatment for psychosis. However, more research needs to be done. Although CBD oil should be safe, THC may not be safe for those with schizophrenia. THC is the psychoactive compound in cannabis; this may increase psychosis for those with schizophrenia.

CBD oil can help fight cancer! Studies have recently shown that CBD oil can be highly valuable in treating cancer. CBD and other compounds in cannabis have the ability to kill tumor cells in colon cancer and leukemia. The CBD reduces human glioma cell invasion and growth, proving it can be an anti-tumor agent. CBD oil has also shown to stop the spreading of cancer cells in cervical cancer.

It is thought that CBD can also be used as a tool in combination therapy for prostate cancer and breast cancer (again, this is due to the CBD's anti-tumor effects). The CBD can also improve the effectiveness of the typical anti-tumor drugs that are being used, and also help with pain reduction.

- CBD can decrease the ability of cancer cells to produce energy – this leads to their death
- CBD treatment helps the LAK (lymphokine-activated killer) cells to kill cancer cells more effectively
- CBD blocks CPR55 signaling which decreases cancer cell proliferation

However, most studies done on CBD oil and cancer are still under what is called "pre-clinical," which means they were not conducted on humans or mammals. It is just important to be mindful of CBD oil having the 100 percent ability to cure cancer.

CBD oil can help stimulate genes and proteins that help break down fat, maintain healthy blood sugar, and increase mitochondria that will help burn calories. Additionally, CBD oil will encourage the body to change white fat to brown fat. White fat is the most common kind of body fat and is the classical form of "fat" we think of. Brown fat is a small fat deposit, and it acts differently than white fat. Brown fat is not considered bad, in fact, it is said to improve health. It improves the body's ability to burn the white fat, regulates blood sugar and creates heat.

Less commonly, CBD oil can reduce the risk of diabetes. A Neuropharmacology study showed that only 32 percent of a group of non-obese, diabetes-prone mice who were given CBD, developed diabetes. In the group of non-obese, diabetes-prone mice that were not given CBD 100 percent of them developed diabetes.

Another less common benefit of CBD oil is its ability to fight multi-drug resistant bacteria. A study done in 2011 showed that CBD oil helped slow the progression of tuberculosis in rats. CBD does not possess antibacterial properties; it inhibits T-cell proliferation. This is important as more and more "superbugs" come about that are antibiotic-resistant, we are running out of options. CBD may be one, powerful option.

In the United States, heart disease is the primary cause of death, and CBD oil can help that. Obviously, leading a healthy lifestyle and eating a healthy diet are most important in combating heart disease, but CBD oil can also be effective. Research has been done that shows that cannabidiol can reduce artery blockage, blood pressure, cholesterol and stress-induced cardiovascular response.

CBD oil can be used as a treatment with Crohn's disease – something that affects 200,000 Americans each year, while in North America, more than half a million people. Crohn's disease is an inflammatory bowel disorder. It causes sores and ulcers in the digestive tract. Symptoms include diarrhea, weight loss, abdominal pain, bloody stools and sometimes skin and eye conditions. It is most common in men ages 15 to 30 and has no cure. Crohn's disease can be treated by managing symptoms with medications, but it is not always so easy. Many of the medications have severely negative side effects that can sometimes be worse than the symptoms that come with having Crohn's disease. The cons associated with traditional Crohn's disease medications include a high rate of addiction (typically associated with opioids).

CBD has the ability to reduce inflammatory hypermotility, which is associated with diseases such as Crohn's. CBD inhibits a liver enzyme that breaks down endocannabinoids, allowing anandamide to exert its natural anti-inflammatory and anti-motility effects.

A study done by the National Institute of Health showed that CBD contains anti-bacterial effects. This is beneficial to those with Crohn's disease, due to how common gastrointestinal infections are.
CBD oil can help your skin! Topical CBD creams can treat many skin conditions like eczema, by encouraging abnormal cell death. CBD can also help with acne by decreasing lipid synthesis and proliferation of human sebaceous glands. CBD also has an anti-inflammatory effect on sebaceous glands, so it has the potential to treat acne vulgaris. CBD oil also reduces the growth of keratinocytes (skin cells), this can help with psoriasis. CBD oil can help regulate the skin's oil production. Vitamin E has always been known to be great for the skin, and CBD oil contains it!

CBD oil helps with oxidative stress, which are the cause of many ailments. Oxidative stress occurs when the body has too many free radicals, and it cannot keep up with neutralizing them. This has become a larger problem more recently, due to our environment being more toxic than it once was.

CBD oil can act as an antioxidant and even has CBD oil is a powerful antioxidant and it even has neuroprotective qualities; in turn, it reduces the damage to neurons caused by the free radicals.

CBD oil can increase appetite, along with relieving vomiting and nausea. This was shown in a study with rats. However, it can be complex, because the CBD helped with vomiting and nausea when the rats were given toxic drugs. When the rats were given high doses of CBD, nausea increased or had no effect.

CBD can bind to cannabinoid receptors in the body, which increase appetite, according to the National Cancer Institute. And for those with food sensitivities, CBD oil helped eliminate them – a small but wonderful improvement in everyday life.

CBD oil has the potential to help one quit smoking, and help with drug withdrawals. A study done by Addictive Behaviors, an international peer journal, showed that smokers who used a CBD inhaler smoked fewer cigarettes throughout the day. The inhaler contained the CBD compound helped curb cravings for nicotine.

Other studies done in the United Kingdom by the University College London had similar results. In this 2013 study, dependent smokers were given a CBD inhaler to use upon having a nicotine craving. It was shown that their cigarette intake reduced by 40 percent. Those dependent smokers who were given a placebo inhaler did not have a significant reduction in their cigarette intake.

A more recent study done in the United Kingdom in May 2018, also showed that those given an 800mg dose of CBD had significant reductions in cigarette cravings.

These studies are significant because they show that CBD oil may be able to help cigarette smokers quit on a few different levels. Cigarette smoking goes beyond being a physical addiction, it is also a habit that has to be broken. Smoking CBD oil could be a similar substitute that actually relieves anxiety.

Using CBD oil as a substitute in place of smoking cigarettes is a great alternative because it is a non-intoxicating compound that does not get you high and actually has a lot of medical benefits.

A study done by Neurotherapeutics showed that CBD can be a good substance for those abusing opioids. CBD has the capabilities to be a good "exit drug." An exit drug has the ability to wean someone off opioids. CBD can do so by helping with the pain that usually, initially, got them addicted to opioids in the first place and by helping with opioid withdrawal symptoms.

A June 2017 study titled, Cannabis As A Substitute For Opioid-Based Pain Medication: Patient Self-Report, where data was collected from nearly 3000 medical cannabis patient, showed that people with access to CBD took fewer prescription opioids for pain. It is also true that doctors prescribe fewer opiates for the pain to people in states that have accessible medical CBD. More obviously, these states also have fewer opioid hospitalizations and fewer overdose deaths.

CBD can help many kinds of recovering addicts. Studies have shown the same, with other substances such as cocaine and alcohol.

A recent Nature study done in March 2018 showed that CBD oil can be successful in treating addiction in animals. Alcohol or cocaine-addicted rats were given CBD oil topically once a day for a week. The rats were then tested to see how they reacted in stressful situations. The research showed that these rats were less likely to relapse, even while in the stressful situations. The study also showed that the rats had reduced impulsivity and anxiety, two traits commonly associated with addiction.

The study went on, to show that the CBD oil had worked on the rats even five months later, even though it was out of their systems. The rats were still less likely to relapse in stressful situations or when provoked by "drug cues" because they had been treated with CBD oil.

CBD oil can even work effectively with animals. Mammals have an endocannabinoid system, just like us humans; therefore, CBD oil can give them the same benefits it gives us.

In cats and dogs CBD oil can help with pain, increasing appetite, getting along with other pets, separation anxiety, excessive crying or barking, and relaxation (maybe for a vet trip).

In order to successfully give your pet CBD oil, you need to find the right dosage for them (just as you'd do with yourself). Start out with a small dosage. A good rule of thumb is 1 milligram for every 10 pounds of their body weight. Eventually, you can level up to 5 milligrams per 10 pounds of body weight. Sometimes you will even have to give a bit more for a more serious condition, such as an excessive pain that your pet is going through. It is recommended to give your pet their CBD oil spread-out, throughout the day – 3-4 times. This is more effective than just giving them one large dose each day.

CBD Oil Benefits Technically Explained

- CBD will activate 5HT1A receptors and 5HT2A receptors (slightly)
- Activating 5HT1A receptors helps with vomiting and nausea, depression, appetite, anxiety, addictions, and sleep
- CBD protects the brain from lack of oxygen - partially via 5HT1A receptors
- CBD increases glucose-dependent insulinotropic peptide.
- CBD takes part in the perception of inflammation and pain by activating the TRPV-1 receptor
- CBD is capable of blocking FAAH enzyme and anandamide reuptake, which indirectly activates CB1 receptors and increases the level of anandamide, making it effective against depression and anxiety
- CBD can reduce seizures by modulating neuron excitability and intracellular Ca^{2+} ions

I hope that you are enjoying reading through this book and that you are finding it helpful. If you wish your thoughts about the book so far, then you can do soi by leaving a review on the Amazon page.

Chapter 3: How to - CBD

There are several ways to consume CBD oil. The four most common ways to consume CBD oil include ingestion (edibles, capsules), sublingual (spray), topical (creams) and inhalation (vaping). The most common of those is ingestion (taking it orally) – you can do this with a concentrated paste or a tincture/drop format. It is important to first hold it under the tongue, so it is absorbed in the mouth. The digestive system breaks some of the CBD down.

It really does not matter what method you choose to take the CBD oil. The objective is simply that the cannabinoids enter your system easily to achieve the results you want. How you take the CBD oil usually relates to how much you are taking, or the "dosage," and how long you want the effects to last.

It seems most people that take CBD oil do not prefer the method most similar to smoking, which is vaping. However, when taking CBD oil by vaping the effects occur quite quicker – within a few minutes, compared to what can be hours.

Additionally, when taking CBD oil in a manner that does not allow the effects to occur until later, the effects often last longer. So it really depends on what you prefer, and are trying to achieve.

If you decide to take CBD oil orally, you will do so by taking capsules, edibles or adding it to the food or drinks you are already consuming. You can also take CBD oil in the form of tincture. You take tincture by placing small drops of it in your mouth, directly under your tongue or adding it to your food or drink. A lot of people prefer a tincture, because of how discreet it is.

CBD oil tinctures sometimes referred to as "drops" come as liquid supplements. They are packaged in a glass bottle with a dropper or spray top to make for easily dispensing. As stated before, the tincture form is very popular. An added factor to that are the ingredients that can be added. Manufacturers often add coconut oil, spearmint, terpenes, essential oils or natural herbs. These all do wonders in masking the potent taste of CBD oil.

When taking CBD oil tincture, use your dropper top to suck up as much CBD oil as desired, and then place it under your tongue. Wait about a minute to a minute in a half to swallow the CBD oil tincture. If the flavor is too much for you, you can try drinking some juice alongside swallowing the CBD oil tincture.

There are many, many types of CBD oil tinctures – varying in flavor, strength, and size. If you do not like one specific kind, think about trying something else before throwing in the towel with tinctures. There truly is something for everyone, when it comes to tinctures.

Some CBD oil is made for vaping pens, which is going to be the method that allows you to feel the effects of the CBD the quickest. When you vape CBD oil, it enters your bloodstream directly through your lungs.

When vaping CBD oil or e-liquid, you will need a vaporizer or vape pen. Buying a vape kit is also an option. A vape kit includes a disposable vape cartridge that will screw into the vaporizer. With a disposable vaporizer pen, you do not have to worry about the hassle of maintaining your vaporizer pen. A regular vaporizer pen will need its tank and coils replaced once in a while. There are many vaping products out there – many of them affordable and disposable!

Vaping CBD oil should not be as harmful as smoking cigarettes. Vaping CBD oil can actually be seen as a sort of relaxing. One CBD oil consumer who vapes said, "When I'm feeling anxious, or in serious need of relaxation, I immediately grab my vaporizer." When you vape, you are inhaling and exhaling. Its two practices many people use to achieve peace and calmness, a bit like performing a type of calming, breathing technique that one may do while meditating or practicing yoga.

Sublingual sprays are also discreet like the tincture form. You can simply spray it under your tongue. The effects of the CBD are also fairly quick.

Topical CBD creams are most effective for those with joint or muscle pain. Topical CBD creams are also popular with those who have inflamed, dry or aging skin. Our skin is actually our largest organ, so topical CBD creams are a great way to properly take care of it through balance and moisturization.

Obviously, topical CBD creams are only to be used externally. You will want to apply them to the target areas – such as where you are in pain, or where your dry skin is located. Using topical CBD creams is super simple. You simply massage the targeted area with the product, much like applying lotion or sunscreen.

Topical CBD creams have anti-inflammatory and pain relieving properties. They can really help those who suffer from arthritis. There are many topical CBD products out there that vary in consistency. Sometimes it is best to try a few out to see what works best for you, and what you hope to achieve with the product.

Another form, in which CBD oil is often consumed, is a pure concentrate. It is a paste-like oil, extracted from the hemp plant. Most likely, your pure concentrate CBD oil will be packaged in an oral syringe, which can be a bit intimidating for some, or may simply be unappealing, but never fear. You do not actually inject the CBD oil.

Squeeze out from the syringe as much CBD oil as you plan to take onto either the back of a spoon, directly under your tongue, or finger. The end result will be placing the CBD oil under your tongue – it is up to you how it gets there!

The reason the CBD oil is placed under the tongue is because, in the mouth, there are capillary glands that absorb the oil. When the capillary glands absorb the CBD oil, it enters your system rapidly. When you swallow the CBD oil, a good amount of it will have already been absorbed by your body.

An average amount of CBD oil to take is about the size of a grain of rice – pretty small! You do not want to over-do it. Better safe, than sorry. So try not to get too much. If anything squeezes less than needed and then you can always squeeze out more.

It is important to be careful during this step because CBD oil when in a pure concentrated form, is a natural oil. Each one is going to vary in its consistency and its flavor. Sometimes the pure concentrate is runny; sometimes it is very thick. If you get something totally dissimilar to what you had before, that is perfectly normal. However, the CBD oil pure concentrate can stain, so be careful when getting it out of the syringe. You do not want to get any on your clothes, floors, or surfaces in your home.

Once the CBD oil pure concentrate is under your tongue, you want to wait a minute or a minute and a half to swallow it. The longer you wait, typically the better the results, this is recommended by most but it really is your call and what you feel most comfortable with.

Be warned that CBD oil does not taste "good." One CBD oil consumer said "pure hemp oil tastes like you grabbed a handful of dirt and grass and ate it. Sometimes it is a little spicy, too." If you simply cannot get over the taste, it is recommended that you take CBD oil sublingually, but it is believed that CBD oil taken in a pure concentrate form is the best way to get a large number of cannabinoids in your system, each day.

One way to get around the "bad" taste of CBD oil in pure concentrate form is to try drinking juice as you swallow it. Apple cider and orange juice seem to be most effective at masking the potent taste of the CBD oil pure concentrate.

As stated before, the CBD oil is going to vary in its consistency and taste due to the harvest. With each harvest will bring a different taste due to terpenes - compounds in the hemp plant. Much like cannabinoids, it is not possible to tell what compounds have formed in the plant until the oil has actually been extracted and then tested. There really is no way to say how a batch will taste until it is already made.

It is hard to know how much CBD oil to take, especially when it is your first time using it. Unfortunately, there is so no standard dosage, and we are all different. The proper dosage for you may not be the proper dosage for everyone else. Our bodies are all very unique, so you are the only one who can adjust your own dosage.

It should also be noted that as of now, there is no scientific information that directs toward how much CBD oil a person should take for something particular. That is how it goes with natural remedies (for now). The FDA allows CBD oil to be sold by manufacturers as a food supplement, not as a type of medicinal product. It will not be until CBD oil is sold as a remedy or medicinal supplement, that we will ever have any scientific data that supports specific dosages.

Since the FDA has to treat CBD oil as a food supplement, it has a type of nutritional label, similar to the ones you see on food items. A requirement of food labels is having a "suggested serving size." Unfortunately, this is a bit of a disservice to consumers of CBD oil since our bodies are all vastly different. The suggested serving size number is arbitrary and should not be regarded, in most cases.

For example, when starting out with CBD oil, it is recommended to start with a smaller dosage. It is important to not simply take a dosage amount you saw online. Use information online as a guide and not as a personalized recommendation. If you are using CBD oil to treat a specific condition, and have a doctor you saw for that condition, then they can give you professional advice regarding CBD oil usage and dosage.

It is very important to think about your current health condition – the severity, your diet and weight, metabolism and if you have a tolerance to CBD already. For example, if your weight changes, your CBD dosage should also change. Metabolism does not typically change as quickly, but lifestyle changes can. If you switch up your activity levels – going from active to sedentary, you will want to think about your CBD dosage. Just remember to take all factors into account. A general rule of thumb is that the heavier you are (physically), the more CBD oil you will have to take. This also applies to the severity of the condition you are trying to treat (the more severe, the more you will have to take).

A general guide for CBD dosage depending on the severity of condition and weight is as follows:

Severity of condition 1 (mild), 2, 3 (medium), 4, 5 (severe)

Weight of person - 31 pounds – 61 pounds: 2mg – 4mg + (1, mild), 4mg – 8mg + (2), 8mg – 12mg + (3, medium), 12mg – 18mg + (4), 18mg – 30mg +(5, severe) Weight of person - 61 pounds - 100 pounds: 4mg - 6mg + (1, mild), 6mg -12mg + (2), 12mg 18mg + (3, medium), 18mg – 24mg + (4), 24mg – 40mg + (5, severe) Weight of person - 100 pounds – 175 pounds: 6mg – 8mg + (1, mild), 8mg – 18mg + (2), 18mg – 24mg + (3, medium), 24mg – 32mg + (4), 32mg – 60mg + (5, severe)

Weight of person - 175 pounds – 250 pounds: 8mg – 10mg + (1, mild), 12mg – 20mg + (2), 22mg – 30mg + (3, medium), 32mg – 40mg + (4), 42mg – 60mg + (5, severe)

When starting out taking CBD oil, make sure to observe the effects – how you feel? It is helpful and recommended, to write down the amount of CBD oil you took, what time, your weight, what you ate that day, how you felt before taking the CBD oil, and how you felt after taking the CBD oil. You can also include anything else you find to be relevant. Make sure to do this every day.

Split up a large dose into a bunch of smaller doses, and take them throughout the day. Do this for a few days to observe the effects and see if it is working for you. You should be able to determine if you need to take less or more. Always do so gradually – take a bit more or a bit less. Large doses can often act as sedatives – making one drowsy, and small doses can act as stimulants – making one alert. You can also experience dizziness, or a dry mouth – these are the most common side effects. The best way to achieve the desired result for you is to simply experiment a little!

Just because CBD is a natural plant extract (there are no dangerous side effects or risk of overdose), does not mean you should take as much as you like. Taking the wrong dosage will not help you with your issue(s) and can make you feel uncomfortable or bad.
On the contrary, there is no data supporting that it is possible to take "too much." A good example is eating fruits and vegetables to improve your health. It is hard to over-do it with something like that. It is not possible to overdose. You might make yourself a bit sick by

overeating, but you will definitely survive. Typically, you are more in trouble when not consuming enough healthy food items (such as fruits and vegetables).

Chapter 4: Possible Side Effects with CBD oil

For the most part CBD oil seems to be misconceived, or simply misunderstood. CBD is mostly considered safe and tolerable. There are a few, minor side effects related to consuming CBD oil.

It is important to remember that CBD oil is not going to cause severe injury or death. It has not been proven to be physically addictive. It is all-natural and in most cases, has been shown to be highly effective and beneficial for those consuming it.

Some of the minor, perhaps unpleasant side effects include:

Dry mouth – Those using CBD oil may experience a dry mouth, which can be a bit unpleasant. This occurs because after consuming CBD oil, the salivary secretion is inhibited by the endocannabinoid system.

A study done in 2006, by Argentinian researchers showed that the cannabinoid receptors (type 1 and type 2), are present in the submandibular glands. The submandibular glands are in charge of producing saliva. When these receptors are activated, it alters salivary production (leading to a dry mouth – this is sometimes referred to as "cotton mouth"). The basis of having a dry mouth is that you are thirsty!

A dry mouth is not that big of a deal at all and can be easily countered. All you have to do is simply consume plenty of hydrating fluids before consuming CBD oil, during and after – or choose one of the three and you will probably be alright. Regardless you are not going to die of a dry mouth, as long as you hydrate at some point in your day. Drinking plenty of water is good for the body and always recommended, regardless if you are consuming CBD oil or not, so again, the possibility of having a dry mouth is not that big of a deal.

Inhibition of hepatic drug metabolism – This occurs alongside decreased activity of p-glycoprotein. CBD oil may also inhibit the activity of cytochrome P450 – some liver enzymes. It is these enzymes that metabolize a good amount of prescription drugs that are used to treat humans. When taken in high doses, the CBD may temporarily make the activity of the P450 enzyme neutral. This will alter the way the drugs metabolize in the body. To explain this more lightly, eating a part of a grapefruit has similar effects on the body, so this may not always be a huge deal. If you are taking prescription drugs, however, it is a good idea to check with a doctor or pharmacist about P450 enzyme activity/reduction before consuming CBD oil or any CBD products.
A list of drugs that interact with CBD

It is important to remember that any drug metabolized by cytochrome P-450 enzymes can possibly interact with CBD.

- Angiotensin II blockers
- Antibiotics
- Anti-psychotics
- Anesthetics
- Anti-depressants
- Anti-epileptics

- Anti-arrhythmias
- Antihistamines
- Benzodiazepines
- Beta-blockers
- Calcium channel blockers
- HIV antivirals
- Immune modulators
- HMG CoA reductase inhibitors
- NSAIDs
- Oral hypoglycemic agents
- PPIs
- Prokinetics
- Steroids
- Sulfonylureas

This list does not include every medication that could potentially be affected by CBD. On the other hand, it is not guaranteed that all of these drugs will have a reaction with CBD use. Therefore it is best to consult your medical professional before consuming CBD oil when under a medication. Also, a doctor can always test to see if your P-450 enzyme system is working correctly, and that your medications are metabolizing correctly.

Drowsiness – This is something that only affects some users of CBD oil, in fact, many people who consume CBD oil say they actually feel more energetic and uplifted after using CBD oil. CBD oil does affect everyone a bit differently. When taking CBD oil in high doses, some will feel drowsy.

Specifically, there are "non-psychoactive" CBD products that contain small amounts of terpenes and cannabinoids. CBD will modulate the effects of both of these, which can cause severe drowsiness – particularly if consumed in doses 60mg+. CBD that is purified to 99.9 percent is considered "mostly" non-psychoactive. However, it is also less effective in this case.

For those who consume CBD oil and feel drowsy, it is just important that they are not operating a motor vehicle for their own safety, and for the safety of others.

Drop in blood pressure – A few studies have shown that after CBD oil consumption (in large doses), there has been a small drop in blood pressure. The issue with this arises in those who have been diagnosed with low blood pressure or take medication for low blood pressure. Low blood pressure can cause one to feel light-headed, which is unpleasant for many. It is advised to consult with a doctor before consuming CBD oil or any CBD products if you do have low blood pressure.

Lightheadedness – Associated with a drop in blood pressure, this is a temporary side effect that can be managed by consuming some form of caffeine prior to consuming CBD oil. Drinking a cup of coffee or tea works great. You will always want to make sure to drink water as well because most caffeinated beverages are typically dehydrating. Again, this is only recommended for people who do not already have low blood pressure.

CBD oil can increases tremors in those with Parkinson's disease. There has been research done showing that when taken in high doses, CBD oil may worsen muscle and tremor movement for those with Parkinson's disease. On the contrary, there has also been a research done, showing that CBD oil is well-tolerated and safe for those with Parkinson's disease. The best advice for someone who has Parkinson's disease and wishes to consume CBD oil is to consume in small doses and consult their doctor first.

Those who have glaucoma should also stay away from CBD oil. CBD oil can exacerbate the ocular pressure that is related to glaucoma.

Adults with epilepsy should also veer from CBD oil products that do not have a significant amount of THC, along with other terpenes/cannabinoids. It has been shown that adult epileptics who consume CBD oil (without sufficient THC) for long periods of time often see their condition worsening. It is different for children with epilepsy because they have not hit puberty yet.

Chapter 5: Is CBD Oil Legal?

CBD oil is not legal in all 50 states. It is legal in 29 states, where medicinal and/or recreational marijuana is legal. Laws regarding the legality of CBD oil typically vary from state to state. In many cases, it has to do with whether the CBD is coming from hemp or marijuana.

According to many in the cannabis industry, as long as the CBD product contains less than 0.3 percent THC, it is classified as hemp under federal law. This means it is legal to distribute and possess. However, state laws on hemp and CBD vary widely.

Several states have passed laws that allow the use of a CBD extract – mostly in oil form, with minimal THC. The CBD oil is often used to treat severe epilepsy in small children. It is important to realize that passing a CBD-specific law is not the same as "legalizing medical marijuana." These CBD-specific laws do not make using the marijuana plant for medical purposes legal.

There are 17 states with CBD-specific laws as of 2018– Georgia, Alabama, Iowa, Indiana, Oklahoma, Kentucky, Missouri, Mississippi, Tennessee, South Carolina, North Carolina, South Dakota, Utah, Wisconsin, Virginia Texas and Wyoming. Each of the states has unique restrictions on use cases and THC levels.

Alabama - "Carly's Law" or SB 174 was signed by Alabama Governor Robert Bentley on April 1, 2014. Carly's Law permits an affirmative protection against prosecution for CBD possession by those suffering from an enervating epileptic condition. Carly's Law says that "a prescription for the possession or use of cannabidiol (CBD) as authorized by this act shall be provided exclusively by the UAB [University of Alabama at Birmingham] Department for a debilitating epileptic condition."

Because marijuana is not federally legal, it is illegal for a doctor to write prescriptions for medical marijuana. Doctors are only allowed to recommend it in the states that have legalized it.

Two years later, another CBD-specific bill was signed into law. On May 4, 2016, HB 61 or "Leni's Law" was signed. This provides favorable justification for the possession of CBD oil "for specified debilitating conditions that produce seizures."

Georgia – "Haleigh's Hope Act" or HB 1 was signed by Georgia Governor Nathan Deal, into law on April 16, 2015. This permits the use of CBD oil that contains not more than 0.5 percent THC for conditions such as Crohn's disease, ALS (Lou Gehrig's disease), seizure disorders, sickle cell anemia cancer, mitochondrial disease, Parkinson's disease and multiple sclerosis.

Governor Deal detailed, "For the families enduring separation and patients suffering pain, the wait is finally over... Now, Georgia children and their families may return home while continuing to receive much-needed care. Patients such as Haleigh Cox, for whom this bill is named, and others suffering from debilitating conditions can now receive the treatment they need, in the place where they belong: Georgia."

Two years later, on May 7, 2018, Governor Deal signed HB 65. HB 65 added intractable pain and PTSD to the list of permitted illnesses for CBD oil use.

Indiana – HB 1148 was signed into law by Indiana Governor Eric Holcomb on April 27, 2017. This law allows the use of CBD that has no more than 0.3 percent THC and at least 0.5 percent CBD for treatment-resistant epilepsy.

The next year in March, Governor Holcomb signed SB 52 into law. SB 52 allows the retail sale of low-THC hemp extract and distribution. Specifically, the low-THC hemp extract has to have a product definition. It has to be derived from cannabis sativa that meets the description of industrial hemp. It cannot contain more than 0.3 percent delta-9-THC. The low-THC hemp extract cannot contain any other controlled substances.

Iowa – SF 2360 was signed by Iowa Governor Terry Branstad on May 30, 2014. Branstad stated of the law, "This bill received tremendous support and truly shows the power of people talking to their legislators and to their governor about important issues to them, to their families and to their children."

Three years later HF 524 was signed by Governor Branstad. HF 524 permits a person to "recommend, possess, use, dispense, deliver, transport, or administer cannabidiol if the recommendation, possession, use, dispensing, delivery, transporting, or administering is in accordance with new chapter 124E of the Iowa Code." This is according to the Iowa Department of Health Office of Medical Cannabidiol website.

The Office of Medical Cannabidiol will issue registration cards to patients in Iowa by December 1, 2018. This law also requires medical cannabidiol dispensaries to begin dispensing by this same date.

Kentucky – SB 124 was signed by Kentucky Kentucky Governor Steve Beshearon April 10, 2014. This law dismisses CBD from the classification of marijuana when it is allotted, transferred or administered pursuant to the inscribed order of a physician working at an associated clinic associated with a Kentucky public university that has a school or college of medicine, or hospital. However, the law does not address how patients may acquire the CBD.

Mississippi – HB 1231 or "Harper Grace's Law" was signed by Mississippi Governor Phil Bryant on April 17, 2014. This law allows for cannabis oil, extract or resin that has more than 15 percent CBD and no more than 0.5 percent THC. Additionally, the CBD oil has to be received from or test by the National Center for Natural Products Research at the University of Mississippi. It also has to be distributed by the Department of Pharmacy Services at the University Of Mississippi Medical Center. This law also offers favorable defense for defendants that suffer from a enervating epileptic disorder and who had accessed the CBD oil in agreement with the requirements that are in the bill. This was effective on July 1, 2014.

Governor Bryant stated of the law, "The bill I signed into law today will help children who suffer from severe seizure disorders. Throughout the legislative process, I insisted on the tightest controls and regulations for this measure, and I have been assured by the Mississippi Bureau of Narcotics that CBD oil is not an intoxicant.

The outcome is a bill that allows this substance to be used therapeutically as is the case for other controlled prescription medications. I remain opposed to any effort that would attempt to legalize marijuana or its derivatives outside of the confines of this bill."

An amendment to the law was signed in by Governor Bryant, a few years later. On March 20, 2017, the amendment allowed the "clarify the use in seizures and other medical conditions," along with allowing other pharmacies, aside from the University of Mississippi Medical Center to dispense CBD (with federal and state regulatory approval).

Missouri – HB 2238 was signed in to law on July 14, 2014, by Missouri Governor Jay Nixon. This permits the use of CBD oil at a minimum of 0.5 percent CBD and is less than 0.3 percent THC. It can be used for intractable epilepsy. In order to be qualified, a neurologist needs to justify that after undergoing three treatment options, the patient did not respond effectively.

Registration cards are issued to patients with a diagnosis (who meet the program's conditions) by the Missouri Hemp Extract Registration Program. These registration cards allow patients to use and possess CBD oil in their state of Missouri.

North Carolina – HB 1220 was signed into law by North Carolina Governor Pat McCrory on July 3, 2014, allowing universities to perform clinical trials using CBD oil that was no more than 0.3 percent THC and has at least 10 percent CBD. The CBD oil could only be for the treatment of intractable epilepsy.

An amendment to the law was made on July 16, 2015. Governor McCrory signed HB 766. The amendment stated that "hemp extract must be composed of less than nine-tenths of one percent (0.9 percent) tetrahydrocannabinol (THC) by weight, at least five percent (5 percent) cannabidiol (CBD) by weight and may contain no other psychoactive substances." This is according to the North Carolina Department of Health and Human Services (DHHS). Only patients are allowed possession and use of CBD oil. It is illegal to produce and cultivate hemp extract in North Carolina. However, those in possession of the DHHS Caregiver Registration letter are allowed to bring hemp extract with them outside their home.

Oklahoma – HB 2152 or "Katie's Law" was put into effect on April 30, 2015, signed by Oklahoma Governor Mary Fallin. This law permits the use of CBD oil that has no more than 0.3 percent THC for the treating severe forms of epilepsy.

Fallin stated, "This bill will help get sick children potentially life-changing medicine. By crafting the legislation in a way that allows for tightly controlled medical studies, we can ensure we are researching possible treatments in a responsible and scientific way. The CBD oil we are studying is a non-intoxicating derivative of marijuana. It is not marijuana, and it is not anything that can make you 'high.' This law has been narrowly crafted to support highly supervised medical trials for children with debilitating seizures. It is not a first step towards legalizing marijuana, and I will never support the legalization of marijuana in Oklahoma."

HB 2835 was signed by Governor Fallin on May 13, 2016. The law added "spasticity due to multiple sclerosis or due to paraplegia, intractable nausea and vomiting, and appetite stimulation with chronic wasting diseases" to approved conditions. It went into effect on July 1, 2016.

Another amendment – HB 1559, was made on April 17, 2017, excluding "any federal Food and Drug Administration-approved cannabidiol drug or substance" from the definition of marijuana. This went into effect on November 1, 2017.

South Carolina – S 1035 or "Julian's Law" was signed by South Carolina Governor Nikki Haley on June 2, 2014. This law, pertaining to anyone who obtains a written and signed certification (by a physician) "stating that the patient has been diagnosed with Lennox-Gastaut Syndrome, Dravet Syndrome, also known as 'severe myoclonic epilepsy of infancy', or any other severe form of epilepsy that is not adequately treated by traditional medical therapies and the physician's conclusion that the patient might benefit from the medical use of cannabidiol."

Patients can use CBD oil that has more than 15 percent CBD and less than 0.9 percent THC. This CBD oil is provided by the Medical University of South Carolina, as a part of their study determining the effects of CBD in help to control seizures.

South Dakota – South Dakota Governor Dennis Daugaard signed SB 95 into law on May 17, 2017. This law added CBD to the already existing list of Schedule IV controlled substances. It also exempted it from the classification of marijuana. The specification was that the CBD must be a product approved by the FDA (United States Food and Drug Administration).

Tennessee – SB 2531 was signed into law on May 16, 2014, by Tennessee Governor Bill Haslam. The law states the CBD oil has to have less than 0.9 percent THC "as part of a clinical research study on the treatment of intractable seizures when supervised by a physician practicing at... a university having a college or school of medicine." The study was approved until 2018 – for four years.

SB 280 was signed into law on May 5, 2015, by Governor Haslam. This allows the use of CBD oil that is less than 0.9 percent THC. The CBD oil has to be obtained outside of Tennessee but obtained legally in the United States. This bill was effective immediately.

Texas – SB 339 was signed on June 1, 2015, by Texas Governor Greg Abbott. This law permits using CBD oil that is not more than 0.5 percent THC and is at least 10 percent CBD for treating intractable epilepsy. It requires patients to get approved by two certified specialists.

Governor Abbot stated, "There is currently no cure for intractable epilepsy, and many patients have had little to no success with currently approved drugs. However, we have seen promising results from CBD oil testing, and with the passage of this legislation, there is now hope for thousands of families who deal with the effects of intractable epilepsy every day."

The law was written to require physicians to prescribe CBD, which is actually illegal in regards to the federal law. States can allow doctors to "recommend" but not "prescribe." Yet, the Texas Compassionate Use Programs says they define prescription as "an entry in the compassionate-use registry." As of December 15,

2017, three dispensing organizations had been licensed.

Utah – HB 105 or "Charlee's Law" was signed by Utah Governor Gary Herbert on March 21, 2014. This law allows the use and possession of marijuana extract for people with intractable epilepsy. They have to have a statement signed by a neurologist. The extract must be less than 0.3 percent tetrahydrocannabinol (THC) and has at least 15 percent of cannabidiol (CBD) by weight. It also cannot have any other psychoactive substance. The law went into effect on July 1, 2014.

The marijuana extract must be received in a sealed container from a laboratory that is licensed in the state in which it was produced. It has to have a label declaring the extract's origin and exact ingredients. Then it must be transported by the laboratory to the Utah Department of Health. It is the Utah Department of Health's job to decide the details of the registration program.

Kristen Stewart of *Salt Lake Tribune* wrote, "HB105 gives Utahns with epilepsy trial access to a non-intoxicating, seizure-stopping cannabis oil. But it does not take effect until July 1, 2014, and until then, Utahns can not legally possess cannabis oil. And obtaining it after that date will still risk violating federal law — and require jumping through a set of still-vaguely defined hoops. Currently, patients will need to travel to states where medical marijuana is legal and import cannabis oil themselves. Doing so remains technically a violation of federal law." This was from her March 25, 2014 article titled "Utah Families Celebrate Passage of Cannabis 'Charlee's Law.'"

In accordance with Utah law, in order to legitimately possess hemp extract, a person must obtain (by application) a hemp extract registration card, given by the Utah Department of Health, Office of Vital Records and Statistics.

Virginia – HB 1445 was signed on February 26, 2015, by Virginia Governor Terry McAuliffe. The law states, "In any prosecution... involving marijuana in the form of cannabidiol oil... it shall be an affirmative defense that the individual possessed such oil pursuant to a valid written certification... for treatment or to alleviate the symptoms of... intractable epilepsy." The CBD oil must have at least 15 percent CBD and no more than 5 percent THC.

Governor McAuliffe stated,"The whole reason I got into politics was to bring about a positive impact in the lives of families across the Commonwealth. This piece of legislation is a tremendous step forward."

Three years later, Governor Ralph Northam signed HB 1251. This generalized the list of conditions to "any diagnosed condition or disease determined by the practitioner to benefit from such use."

A process is being implemented by the Virginia Board of Pharmacy that issues pharmaceutical processor permits for CBD oil. It was anticipated that this RFA (Request for Application) process would be open in spring 2018.

Wisconsin – AB 726 or "Lydia's Law" was signed on April 16, 2014, by Wisconsin Governor Scott Walker. The law states "any physician may provide an individual with a hard copy of a letter or other official documentation stating that the individual possesses cannabidiol to treat a seizure disorder if the cannabidiol is in a form without a psychoactive effect." A Governor's office release stated that the law was "clearing the way for a new treatment for children suffering from seizure disorders, pending FDA approval."

SB 10 was signed into law by Governor Scott Walker on April 17, 2017. This law simplified the law by moving "seizure disorder" to "medical condition."

Wyoming –HB 32 became effective on July 1, 2015. Wyoming Governor Matt Mead didn't sign the bill or veto it. This allowed the use of hemp extract that has at least 15 percent CBD and no more than 0.3 percent THC, only to be used for the treatment of intractable epilepsy.

As stated by the Wyoming Department of Agriculture (WDA), "We do not anticipate a licensing program prior to the start of 2019... The main hurdle the program faces is funding... This legislation had no appropriation attached, and in order to start the new program, the WDA needs funding to start and implement the program."

Whether or not CBD oil is legal in regards to where you live is something you will have to look up and do your own research with. I recommend using online resources such as your state's government website if it is unclear. If you are fortunate enough to live in a state where recreational marijuana is legal - Alaska, Colorado,California, Maine,Oregon, Nevada,Massachusetts, Vermont, Washington and Washington DC - finding CBD oil products can be as simple as a doing a quick Google search such as "CBD oil near me."

In states such as Oregon, finding CBD oil could be as simple as walking down the street if you are living in a large city such as Portland, where dispensaries are conveniently located on nearly every block. Dispensary workers or "budtenders" are knowledgeable when it comes to cannabis – they know their stuff! If you simply tell them what you are looking for, or what you hope to achieve, they should be able to lead you in the right direction. They can also tell you the amount of CBD in the oil and the amount of THC (if any). These two things will also be listed on the product.

Chapter 6: Where to Buy CBD Oil/Costs

CBD oil can be purchased from many different places including dispensaries, online, herbalist shops, co-ops, dispensaries and more. CBD oil products are either made from marijuana or hemp plants.

It is important to know what exactly it is that you are looking for before purchasing. This will help your search, and as far as where to get the CBD oil.

Some of the most popular and highly rated websites to buy CBD oil off of include:

CBDistillery is said to be the "best full spectrum." CBDistillery sells excellent quality CBD that is also fairly priced. 5000mg full spectrum CBD oil will cost you $.05/mg. Many also say that their CBD oil has a pleasant taste as well!

CBDistillery offers free shipping on domestic orders over $75 USD. They sell it in tincture form, isolate powder and slab, capsules, and much more. CBDistillery has a very large inventory of products. Their prices range from as low as $5 USD to $400 USD.

Lazarus Naturals is said to have the best value. This company has the ability to get CBD oil to large amounts for people on a budget. Their oil is said to not taste the best, but you have to remember it is also priced at $.04/mg.

Their products typically range in price from $15 USD to $200 USD. Lazarus Naturals appears to have more products for sale than most of the highly rated CBD oil websites. They sell tinctures, capsules, isolates, pet products, coconut oil, and more.

4 Corners Cannabis is known for being the highest quality when it comes to getting help with medical issues. 4 Corners Cannabis is a bit expensive however at $.20/mg.

Their products typically range from $40 USD to $200 USD. They have a $5 USD flat fee shipping rate, and all orders are processed within 24 hours. Their items for sale include salve, vape oil, tincture and even clothing.

Kat's Naturals is the best THC free CBD oil. For those specifically looking for zero THC, Kat's Naturals is for you. Although most CBD oils have a very small amount of THC, leading to a more noticeable ammount of THC Kat's Natural's CBD products are also known to taste good.
Kat's Natural is a bit of a different website set up. They offer five day, two week or one-month trials on their products.

Canna Trading Co. is going to have the best CBD oil for anxiety and for sleep! Canna Trading Co. will even formulate for your specific ailment. The company adds terpenes to their CBD to make an anti-anxiety remedy that is truly effective. Canna Trading Co. has also created a CBD oil that will put you right to sleep and eliminates any drowsy feelings when you wake up.

Their products tend to range from $16 USD to $110 USD. Canna Trading Co. sells vaporizer pens, tinctures, CBD capsules and more, even clothing.

Pure Kana has one of the best CBD oils for pain relief. This company has helped thousands of patients around the United States. Pure Kana has been in the news and in features in High Times and HERB.

Pure Kana is a unique company because of their CO_2 extraction process – which is rather unique. Their process results in nearly 99 percent pure CBD oil. Their CBD oil has no flavor but is a nutritional and dietary supplement to help with vitality and health. It has been shown to treat inflammation, anxiety, sleeping issues, chronic pain, and swelling.

Pure Kana's CBD oil is organic, non-GMO, third-party, laboratory-tested (ensuring potency and safety), and has no herbicides, solvents, chemical fertilizers or pesticides.

Plus Pure Kana frequently runs promos and specials through their website. They deliver all throughout the United States. Prices range from $48 USD to $139 USD.

VerifiedCBD is another good choice when it comes to CBD oil. Although their products are made in Florida, they are more of a global company and sell CBD oil in more than 50 different countries. HuffPost, the Guardian, and the Washington Post have all raved about Verified CBD.

Customers love Verified CBD due to the purity of their product and how you can buy it directly. They have a return customer rate of 71 percent.

Another thing customer's love about Verified CBD is their environmental integrity. The production of over the counter and synthetic medications often heavily pollutes the environment, along with having toxic effects on the human body and negative side effects!

Verified CBD is committed to not doing any of this. They produce their product without damaging the ozone layer. They do not use poisonous chemicals in order to improve the flavor, and their products are biodegradable. Verified CBD also practices good manufacturing practices (GMP).

They sell capsules, oils, sprays, pet products and more. Verified CBD also runs frequent specials – there's a good chance the product you are interested in has been heavily discounted!

The best CBD oils for pets include Pet Health CBD (best overall and most affordable), Lazarus Naturals (best new entry), Kat's Naturals (best isolate) and 4 Corners Cannabis (best quality).

Pet Health CBD is typically going to be the most popular among people. They have products such as anti-separation CBD, coconut oil and CBD oil tincture, daily wellness CBD capsules, muscle and joint CBD coconut oil, and CBD tincture. Their products range from $39 USD to $50 USD.

Most of these websites run specials, and if you do a quick Google search, you can usually find some type of "offer code" that will give you a percentage off of your product.

Other popular and highly rated websites to buy CBD oil from include: **Receptra, CBDfx, Sagely Naturals, Endeca, American Shaman, Pure Spectrum, Mana Artisan Botanics and NuLeaf Naturals.**

Where you purchase your CBD oil is entirely up to you! There are thousands of websites selling the product, and as you will be the one consuming it, it is best for you to do your own research and decide what it is that you want and need. The sites listed above have simply been my recommendations and can be used as a basic starting point.

Before making your purchase, you may want to check again into the laws in your state regarding CBD oil. Although somewhat unlikely, you would hate to get into any kind of legal trouble by simply purchasing something as harmless as CBD oil.

Chapter 7: Success Stories Related to CBD

Charlotte, Colorado Springs, Colorado – Dravet syndrome

Charlotte, at just six years old, was living with Dravet syndrome, which is a form of epilepsy that is not treatable with typical epilepsy medications. Doctors had all but basically given up. Charlotte's parents did not know what to do, or where to turn. Fortunately, Charlotte's father saw a video online of a boy who was treated with cannabis for his Dravet syndrome. Charlotte's parents applied for a medical marijuana card for their daughter, making her the youngest person in Colorado to ever get one. The CBD treatment was highly effective for Charlotte. Even leading to a strain of cannabis being named, "Charlotte's Web."

Angie, Omaha, Nebraska – Bladder Cancer

Angie was diagnosed with stage three bladder cancer at the age of 75. Fortunately for Angie, she had spent most of her life relatively healthy. The bladder cancer changed everything, however. Angie was prescribed boat-loads of medications and had chemotherapy for a total of nine months. Coming out of the chemo, Angie's bladder did not work at all anymore, but she was thankful to still be alive.

Angie was in a lot of pain and was just generally unwell, that was when her daughter, Kit, mentioned

CBD oil. Angie takes about 15 drops of CBD oil each day – some at night and some in the morning. She said CBD oil has boosted her immune system, gives her energy and helps a lot with the pain she is in. Kit comments on how active her mother is, once again. Even the doctors that treated Angie for her bladder cancer say that they are surprised she is still alive, and recommend that she keeps doing whatever it is that she is doing.

Ben, Baltimore, Maryland - PTSD, Anxiety, Diabetes

Ben, a U.S. Army veteran suffered from PTSD due to several deployments with the Army, along with being diagnosed with diabetes and anxiety later in life. It is likely the diabetes was brought on by a poor diet and becoming overweight, something Ben says was related to his PTSD. One way of coping for him was overeating, and then being too depressed to exercise, or lead an active lifestyle.

When Ben was around 50 years old, he decided to try to get help for his issues. Unfortunately, the doctors just gave him a bunch of pills that did not really help with his conditions, they just masked them temporarily. Each day, Ben was taking around 10 different prescription medications. Ben, going into it, was optimistic, hopeful that something would "cure" him. However, these pill concoctions never did that for him.

When Ben's wife, Alice, began living a healthier, more organic lifestyle, this began to get the ball rolling with holistic alternatives. Alice started to cook organically, removed sugar from their diets and got into essential oils. Ben following suit with his wife's new lifestyle, started to research CBD oil. Ben did his research and found a product that worked for him.

He started by taking 5-8 drops of CBD oil, and the results were nearly instantaneous. Prior to taking CBD oil, it was hard for Ben to be around his large family as a group, including his grandchildren. Having that many people in one space caused him great anxiety and triggered his PTSD. Ben says he actually enjoys the time with his family now and looks forward to being around them.

The CBD oil also helped greatly with a lot of his diabetes symptoms. Ben feels so much more at peace and at ease since beginning to take CBD oil.

Reese, Portland, Oregon – Broken neck and dislocated ankle

Reese, at 17 years of age, was in a horrendous car accident leaving her with a broken neck. Although the injury was over 20 years ago, for Reese, she has suffered from chronic pain due to the injury since it happened. Recently, Reese also dislocated her ankle, which has made the chronic pain throughout her body even worse.

Being in so much constant pain has made Reese unable to sleep, and in turn, unable to work at her job as a public school teacher. Reese felt as if her life was in shambles and did not know what to do. Fortunately for her, a friend recommended CBD oil. Reese did some research and ordered some online.

Nowadays Reese is taking about 20 drops of CBD oil a day. She says it helps her sleep through the night and relaxes her in a way she has never felt before. The CBD oil also improves her mood. For the first time since her car accident – 20 years ago – Reese feels energetic.

The best part of it all, according to Reese, is that she has even been able to return to her a job as a public school teacher. "CBD oil changed my life for the better. I had started to lose hope completely. I didn't think I'd ever not be in pain. I had essentially thrown in the towel and was falling into a deep hole of despair and depression. CBD oil pulled me out. It gave me a life worth living," she says.

Melody, Fairbanks, Alaska – Chronic back pain

Melody has had chronic back pain since a work-related injury 20 years ago. Now at 70, she is retired but still in constant pain. Pain so bad that she has lost her appetite. Melody could feel herself getting weaker and weaker due to the inability of being able to eat.

The doctors prescribed Melody Fentanyl, a highly addictive opioid. Some of the side effects of opioids include headaches, lightheadedness, dizziness and gastrointestinal issues. Melody's body was heavily reliant on the Fentanyl, along with building up quite a tolerance.

However, instead of taking more and more Fentanyl, Melody decided she wanted to try something new, something different. Melody wanted to experiment with something more natural and not highly addictive. Melody began taking CBD oil each day, and her appetite almost instantly returned.

Melody could finally eat again and noticed her body start to become stronger. The CBD oil also relieved a lot of her pain and gave her a newfound energy she had not felt in years.

Derek, Raleigh, North Carolina –Chronic pain

Derek spent all of his adolescence and young adult life participating in extreme sports like skiing, waterskiing, dirt motorbiking, and more. Unfortunately, many people who participate in these types of sports are highly susceptible to injury. At one point Derek hurt his knee dirt biking and had to have surgery requiring him to take pain relievers for the pain. A few years later, Derek broke his ankle skiing. A few more years after that, he broke his ribs while he was motorbiking. What is miraculous is that none of these injuries ever scared Derek from returning back to doing what he loves – doing extreme sports. The downside is he was pretty messed up, physically.

By the time Derek was middle-aged, he was constantly in a lot of pain, mostly in his back area. After going to the doctor and having an MRI, it was discovered that Derek had seven bad disks in his back, which went up from his spine to his neck.

Derek had a procedure done that burns the nerves. However, he was still in a lot of pain and being prescribed more medications such as highly addictive opiates. Fortunately for Derek, he never got addicted, which cannot be said for many who are prescribed the same drugs. He took the drugs for 10 years to manage his pain and continue his job, working as a plumber.

Derek had mixed feelings about the pain relievers from the beginning but was not sure what other option he had. Eventually, he decided he was going to get off the medications. Derek began to get the feeling that the doctors and people he was working with to manage his pain, were not really interested in helping him get better, or what was best for him. He felt like all they wanted to do was make money, by pushing the pain medicines on him.

Derek first tried vaping marijuana in concentrate form in 2015. He had recently decided to stop taking the pain medications and was having some withdrawals. At first, Derek smoked THC, but after doing his research, he got into CBD and realized that was exactly what he needed.

Since beginning to use CBD oil with a vaporizer, Derek has felt fantastic. His muscle and joint pain have severely reduced. He started out taking 10 drops of CBD – 5 in the morning and 5 in the evening. Nowadays – three years later, he takes about 15 drops, three times a day.

Derek says that he feels even better than he did while taking those highly addictive pain relievers. The best part is that CBD oil is natural, it comes from the earth, it is not physically addictive like the prescription medications he was taking, and it is actually a lot less expensive! In the long run, Derek believes his health will be much better, and he strongly believes he made the right choice discontinuing his medication use and switching to CBD oil.

Jackie, at two years of age, had suffered from several kinds of seizures since she was just five months old. She was prescribed over 12 different kinds of over the counter medications such as Klonopin and Depakote - these simply did not work. They also had horrible side effects. Of course, Jackie's parents were devastated but were determined to never give up on their daughter. They began doing some research. They discovered CBD oil but it was not legal yet in the state where they lived, so in order to get Jackie the help she needed, they temporarily moved to a motel in Colorado.

Once in Colorado, Jackie's parents began giving her CBD oil. Since being treated with CBD oil, Jackie's seizures have reduced by over 90 percent. CBD oil also has no negative side effects on Jackie, unlike the prescription medications she was given. CBD oil has also given Jackie the ability to get off those pharmaceutical medications.

Brandon, at the age of two, was diagnosed with leukemia. His leukemia was particularly aggressive – doctors said he only had an eight percent chance of surviving.

Brandon was on chemotherapy that made his tiny, two-year-old body extremely ill. He had nerve damage in his legs, was in massive amounts of pain and even went almost a month without being able to eat.

As a final attempt to save Brandon's life, his mother decided to treat him with CBD oil. After just a few weeks of CBD oil treatment, Brandon's condition improved greatly. He even went into remission shortly after.

Today, Brandon is five years old and doing great, despite doctors stating it was almost certain his leukemia would return.

Collin, at 16, was diagnosed with Crohn's disease. Unfortunately, his Crohn's disease was very severe - stunting his growth and causing him to be in severe pain. Medications were simply not working. Collin's family decided, in order to try to save Collin, they would move to Colorado where the CBD oil Collin needed, was legal. In just a few months Collin's symptoms nearly went away, and he had put the weight that he greatly needed.

Prior to his treatment, Collin had numerous ulcers and inflammation in his colon. In a little over a year, the ulcers and inflammation were gone. Collin is currently doing great and finally able to enjoy all the teenage activities he once dreamed of.

Susie was diagnosed with optic pathway glioma at the age of just one. Doctors said that the tumor would not do well with chemotherapy and it was best to just try to make sure the tumor didn't grow. That was not good enough for Susie's parents, however, and rightfully so.

After using a combination of CBD-oil and high-THC, the tumor is now almost completely gone. And, even though doctor's said Susie would most likely go blind in her left eye, she never has!

Cindy, a resident of Australia, was diagnosed with Stage IV non-small lung cancer at the age of 35, in 2014. She was told her cancer was terminal and was given perhaps 6 to 9 months to live if she got on a medication called Tarceva. Thankfully, Cindy did her research and decided to give CBD oil a try. Upon taking CBD oil alongside the Tarceva, Cindy went into remission that very same year.

Unfortunately, Cindy's cancer returned the following year. However, this time the tumors were much smaller than the original and Cindy is determined to beat cancer once again, with a more aggressive CBD oil therapy approach. She is certain she can beat it again, and that is all thanks to CBD oil.

Shelley had a traumatic brain injury, and a concussion five years ago that caused her to have headaches. Once she began taking CBD oil, the headaches stopped. Along with ridding her of headaches, CBD oil also helped Shelley with anxiety and concentration.

David has multiple sclerosis – some of his symptoms included headaches, insomnia, spasms, and fatigue. CBD oil has greatly helped with all of these symptoms. David feels better than he has in ages and is full of energy.

Keith had two strokes in the past four years and was diagnosed with rheumatoid arthritis, causing him pain and lethargy. CBD oil has allowed Keith to get off a lot of the prescription drugs he once was on and has helped a lot with his pain. Keith says he almost feels better than he ever did before he was diagnosed with rheumatoid arthritis. CBD oil has truly changed his life.

Lisa was diagnosed with CVID (Common Variable Immune Deficiency) – a rare primary immunodeficiency disease, two and a half years ago. Shortly after being diagnosed with CVID, Lisa was also diagnosed with leukemia. These two diagnoses combined with migraines and put Lisa in a lot of pain. Upon taking CBD oil, Lisa began to feel great relief after just a few weeks. CBD oil also helped Lisa get off a lot of her prescription medications.

Alyssa has dealt with panic attacks and anxiety all of her life. Unfortunately, as she'd gotten older they'd only gotten worse. After feeling like she had tried everything, Alyssa decided to give CBD oil a try. Alyssa says for the first time, she has started to feel "normal," thanks to CBD oil.

Noah had four herniated disks in his back, caused by a work accident. He was barely able to move, taking many medications such as morphine and OxyContin – a prescription drug as addictive, and strong as heroin. After starting to take CBD oil, Noah has seen a significant reduction in the pain he was in and was even able to stop taking the highly addictive OxyContin.

Kendra sliced her hand open with a beer bottle while working as a bartender. The cut severed her medial nerve and caused her a great deal of pain. CBD oil has also allowed Kendra to get off addictive prescription medications she was taking before.

Steven has a chronic skin disorder called Hailey-Hailey. The disorder causes painful blisters, inflammation, and rashes. Using CBD oil topically helps Steven manage his disorder more effectively than ever.

Conclusion

At this point, you should feel very comfortable and knowledgeable about CBD oil. We have discussed what it is/where it comes from – the science behind what it does to your body, and the many, many health benefits associated with CBD oil (like pain relief and help with epilepsy). Hopefully, you feel ensured about whether CBD oil is right for you or not. You may even feel like a CBD oil expert!

We looked at the various ways to consume CBD oil, how to do so properly and how to achieve your desired results (like vaping CBD oil for the quickest results). You should feel confident in your own ability to consume CBD oil, in whichever way that works best for you! There is no one size fits all with CBD oil.

You should feel versed on any negative side effects associated with CBD oil. Although there does not seem to be too many, CBD oil may cause problems for those with pre-existing conditions such as Parkinson's disease. We looked at all the complex legality issues with CBD oil, and how they vary from state to state. No one should be going to jail over CBD oil! I showed you where to pick up your own CBD oil – which websites have the best product, which websites have the best value, and what it is that all these websites have to offer. Lastly, we learned about several real-life people, with their own real-life success stories that have to do with CBD oil. These inspiring stories are a great segue for you to have your own CBD oil success story. Good luck and happy healing!

I hope you enjoyed reading through this book and that you found it helpful. If you wish to leave a review, then you can do so on the Amazon page.

CPSIA information can be obtained
at www.ICGtesting.com
Printed in the USA
LVHW031035120423
744157LV00010B/91